I0438424

The Ultimate Guide To Become An Early Riser For Life

How To Awake Early And Be Productive Forever

John K.

Table of Contents

Introduction

Early to bed and early to rise, makes a man healthy, wealthy, and wise.

-Benjamin Franklin

I want to thank you and congratulate you for purchasing the book, "The Ultimate Guide to Become an Early Riser for Life."

This book contains proven steps and strategies on how to improve your productivity by waking up early. Proven to be an effective way to boost your creativity and planning ability, waking up early has been the secret to success by some people who are now known throughout the world. Whether you are a student, a professional, a full-time mother, or a freelancer trying to balance everything in your life, this book would definitely help you become more productive.

This book provides helpful information, effective tips, and step-by-step ways on how to become an early riser and increase your success rate. In this world where everyone seems to be preoccupied with a lot of things that even 24 hours seem to short, being an early riser would definitely give you an extra edge to function well and become more efficient.

Here's a fact: some of the greatest people that the world has known are early risers. Aristotle, Thomas Jefferson, and Benjamin Franklin, to name a few, are certified early risers. Thomas Jefferson, for instance, once said, 'The sun has not caught me in bed for fifty years." This statement alone obviously implies that he is an early riser. He usually wakes up at 5am in the morning to have some coffee, smoke his pipe, and plan his day.

Jefferson, among many other successful people in this world, is an early riser and achiever. Early risers achieved many things in life because they have plenty of time to do it. And guess what? You can be as productive as them, too. With this book in hand, you'll have full access to tips that would help you become an early riser starting today.

Here's a preview of what you'll read inside:

- Knowing the point of becoming an early riser

- The Sweet Perks of rising early

- Getting a good sleep

- Things to do to keep yourself awake

- Forming habits of becoming an early riser

All these information awaits you. So, read on and become an early riser. Thanks again for purchasing this book, I hope you enjoy it!

Chapter 1 – Knowing the Point of Becoming an Early Riser

Being excited about waking up early is understandable. However, before you delve into the 'steps' on becoming an early worm, there are things that you need to know first. And this chapter covers important things so you can be successful on becoming an early riser.

To be able to make a difference in your life, and do things well, it is important that you know where you are in your life right now. You should know in what point in your life are you shifting from or where you are in this journey. This is to help you draw a clear path to where you're headed. Know that assessing where you are in life is an integral part before starting anything massive. Yes, anything.

For you to be successful in making a shift or a change in your life, you must be clear about certain things first. And for you to do this, you can follow these simple steps:

1. **Clear your mind**

Most of us make drastic changes out of excitement or out of curiosity. Well, those reasons won't do when you want to become more productive. Changing a habit or a lifestyle would greatly affect your life and would define your life which means that you need to think things carefully before making any move. Clearing your mind would help you focus on the change that you want to happen therefore would you to start fresh and motivated. A clear mind can make way for clear visions of your goals.

2. Identify the 'points' of doing something

In everything you do, you should have a clear purpose in doing it. In making a change or shift of direction, you have to know where you will go. Therefore, you should identify the 'points' in making big changes.

You should know the 'point' of doing this change. What's the point of becoming an early riser? Why are you going to make this change? What do you want to achieve? Ask yourself these questions for they are vital for you to have a clear goal in doing things. Goals are important so you'll have a driving force to finish something. And more importantly, identify which 'point' you are going. Know where you are headed or where you want to go in life. Identify the points so you'll be guided and not get lost in the process.

3. Recognize your blockages and overcome them

Recognize what hindrances would inhibit you from becoming an early riser. Blockages can be mental or emotional blockages that can affect you from achieving something. Here are the most common blockages that might get in your way from becoming an early riser.

- Not a morning person – schedules or habits are the definite reasons why someone is not a morning person. People who cannot wake up early are usually those who are working in a night shift. There are also those people who are used to sleeping late at night because they have formed the habit of doing so. Not being a morning person shouldn't stop your from changing your lifestyle or habit. However, let this be clear to everyone that although waking up early helps in increasing your productivity, this may not work for everyone. There are people who work best during the night and not adapting this habit of waking up early is totally fine.

- Laziness – perhaps this is one of the most common reasons why many people can't get up early in the morning. It is understandable that some people would want to stay in the comfort of their crisp sheet and sleep more. However, doing so won't help you become more productive. Therefore you should learn to get rid of laziness and start getting out of bed earlier that you usually do.

- Not motivated enough – everyone needs that reason to get up every cold morning, and if you don't have one, you must create one. A motivation can be anything you want to achieve that can be achieved only when you wake up early morning. Perhaps you want to have more time to plan your day, or you want to see the sun rise, it could be anything you can think of.

After you have carefully assessed yourself and finally gotten over the important things mentioned above then you are ready to start the course. If you have cleared your mind, and identified your goals then buckle up and become an early riser with the helpful tips presented in the next chapters.

Chapter 2 – The Sweet Perks of Waking Up Early

For you to be more motivated to become an early riser, it is best to know what you can get out of waking up early. Nothing pushes people to do something than the rewards or perks they get out of doing something. So, to fuel your journey, here are the sweet perks that you can get out of waking up earlier than the sun.

1) Expand productivity

When you wake up early, you can start things early as well and that would mean getting things done ahead of your allotted time or you can have time for more work. Waking up early gives you time to organize your work and plan your day ahead. You can have time to think of yesterdays work and assess your performance. With that enough thinking, you can come up with plans and strategies for improvement. With an organized schedule and a focused mind, you are sure to finish more tasks in an organized manner plus you can have the energy and time to do some extra work.

2) Avoid Cramming or morning anxiety

If you wake up with plenty of time to get things done then there's no need to cram. Waking up early can provide you plenty of time to check your emails, double check the proposal or project you are going to submit, or practice your speech if you are going to give one later in the day.

3) Enjoy the Stillness

Early mornings are the best time to enjoy the stillness of the surroundings. That stillness is rare during the day when everyone is busy at work or you are in a traffic jam. Having a time of solitude would keep your mind clear and focused.

4) Increase your creativity

During early mornings, your mind is focused which means that it is the perfect time to think of creative things. Take advantage of the quietness of early mornings to come up with the best ideas you cannot think of during busy office hours or noisy environment at work.

5) Improve your health

With some spare time in the morning, you can have time to take a walk or run around your neighborhood. Be active or hit the gym. Early mornings are the best time to exercise or do some runs when the sun is not too hot and the air is fresh. Compared to waking up late and immediately hitting the shower, you have more time to listen to your body and keep it healthy when you wake up early.

6) More time to reflect

The calmness of the environment lets you think and reflect. No one will disturb you during this early hour so why meditate or write down the things you've wanted to write about. With some extra time in the morning, you will be able to visualize your day and be grounded.

7) Counteracting depression

When you have more time to organize your work and think about the things that bother you, you can certainly come up with solutions to your problems. And early mornings can definitely help you with that. Moreover, it is also believed that rising early gets rid of negative energies that contribute to formation of depressing thoughts. So, get up early and shake off those negative vibes that might depress you.

8) More time with Family

Early mornings can be the best time to eat with your kids and spouse. You can eat breakfast with them and talk about everything. Not everyone can do this due to busy schedules. But with that extra time you have, bonding with family in the morning can happen.

Chapter 3 – The Preparation Phase: Getting a Good Sleep

To become an early riser, you need to practice having a good night sleep every night. If you are properly rested and slept enough, your energy level when you wake up would be exceptional. So, it is just right that the first phase to becoming an early riser has something to do with getting better sleep every night.

Here are helpful tips to get you started with the preparation phase to become an early riser.

Keep your clean room

Before you do anything or practice anything that would help you wake up early in the morning, it's best to keep your room tidy. If your bedroom is messy and untidy, your mind is most likely to become just like it. Therefore, it is highly suggested that you keep your room clean and tidy to have a clear and relaxed mind before going to bed. Having a clean environment to sleep in keeps your mind calm and allows you to sleep soundly.

Adjust the lighting

When you are trying to get a good night's sleep, a proper lighting is necessary. Your room's lighting can make a difference in your attempt to get a good sleep. Lights or lamps that are too bright could be confused as sunlight which can inhibit sleep. So, adjust your lighting into a dimmer one or completely turn it off when you decide to sleep.

No coffee and no Booze

Obviously a shot of any alcoholic drinks before sleeping won't help you wake up early. In fact, it might give you a really bad hangover that would make you stay in bed half of the day. Furthermore, drinking coffee before you sleep is another no-no if you want to become an early riser. Coffee contains caffeine, if you don't know yet, and this substance can keep your brain alert. Therefore, coffee prior to sleeping won't help you sleep early.

Do not eat large meals before sleeping

It would be best to avoid eating meals before sleeping as the rush of flavors would definitely keep you awake. Not only that large meals before bed is bad for you waistline, it is also not good for your health because of the slow digestion while sleeping. You will find it hard to sleep when your stomach is still working.

List down the Reasons to wake up early

For you to be more motivated to wake up early the next day, you need to list the important things that you need to do. Listing down your urgent projects would encourage you to wake early so you'll be able to start doing the things you have planned.

No laptops or gadgets in bed

Before you sleep, get rid of any gadgets that you have. Whether it's a laptop or ipod, do not use any of those gadget before sleeping. Even your mobile phones should be far away from you as any of these might disturb you while you are in your deep sleep.

Read a good book

Curl up with a good book prior to sleeping. This would get your mind off things and would definitely empty your mind from stress you experienced thewhole day. Reading would help you relax and can give you a good night's sleep.

Avoid strenuous activities

If you exercise before going to bed, there is a less chance of going to bed early. When your energy is still high and upbeat, your body cannot induce sleep because it needs to relax first and stabilize the system. You cannot sleep with an increased hear rate and high temperature. Therefore, if you want to exercise so you'll feel tired, do it 5 hours before your schedule time of sleeping.

Keep your alarm clock far from you

Although this does not contribute in the quality of your sleep, keeping your alarm clock far from you would help you get up the next morning. If you are using an alarm clock to help you to wake up early, then you better keep it out of your reach. If you place your alarm clock in your bedside table, chances are you would just turn it off or hit the snooze quickly without even thinking about it. By keeping it far from you, you'll definitely get up just to silence it. And that's exactly the point of keeping it far from you: to awake you and help you get up from bed.

No watching of television or Laptop an hour before sleep

Watching of the television or laptop keeps your eyes in active state hence it's suggested that if you plan to go to sleep at a particular time then stop watching television or working on your computer before 1 hour.

Although these things do not contribute to keeping you awake in the morning, they would give you a good night sleep which is important to have high energy when you wake up in the next day.

Chapter 4 – Easy ways to keep you awake

One of the most difficult things when you are still new in becoming an early riser is to keep yourself awake in the morning. Most people who are not used to waking up early find it really tempting to go back to bed and continue their sleep. While it is normal that you feel tired or sluggish when you wake up, going back to sleep won't do you any good.

And to avoid going back to sleep, here are some helpful tips that would definitely keep your senses awake.

1) **Open the Window**

   When you just woke up, your mind and system is most likely not awake yet. So to stimulate your system and awaken your mind, open your window and breathe in fresh air. Take in 5-10 breaths of fresh air and feel your system starting to awaken.

2) **Drink water**

After more than 5 hours of sleeping, your body needs water to hydrate itself and a glass of water would definitely suffice. Drinking water will not only awaken your system but the trip to the fridge would keep you from going back to bed.

3) Walk around

Another method to keep you fully awake is by walking around your room or going outside your house. Look at your surroundings, appreciate the quietness of your environment, and walk around to keep your body moving. Aside from keeping you awake, walking has health benefits to the body. It keeps your muscles strong, your blood flowing, and your mind alert.

4) Meditate

What better way to start your day than to reflect and be grounded for a little while. Early mornings are the best time to meditate. With no noise that will disturb you, you are confident that you can meditate without anyone or anything to interrupt your peaceful moment alone. Meditation can awaken your subconscious mind, helps your dig out creative ideas, and makes your mind work.

5) **Write or finish your artwork**

Whether you are writing a story or painting something, do something that would keep your mind working. These activities are best to keep your mind busy and alert in the morning.

Most people who are still adjusting to the changes needed to become an early riser find it hard to keep their selves awake when getting up. That is understandable which is why these suggestions are listed here to help you overcome that temptation of going back to bed.

Chapter 5 – Forming the Habit

Becoming an early riser doesn't happen overnight or after one attempt. You won't become one if you'd only wake up early every weekend or 3 times a week. To be an early riser, you should wake up early every morning. Yes, it should be done daily so you can form a habit. Here are few important things that you need to remember to be successful in this change that you want to happen in your life.

Be consistent

For you to form the habit of waking up early in the morning, you need to be consistent in waking up early and doing your morning routine. Consistency is always the key to become successful in every change that you want to happen in your life. Although this change needs some sacrifice and requires effort, you are sure to harvest everything you invested on it. Furthermore, consistency also means sleeping in the same time and waking up at the same time as well. This will help your body adopt to change. Being consistent would also make your body familiar with the time you sleep and wake up making it easier for you to rise early in the next morning.

Reward yourself

Reward yourself for every achievement that you fulfill. Don't think that waking up early is always about work and having more time to/for work. Make this change rewarding so you'll be motivated to keep doing it. Buy your favorite book, watch a movie, or eat in an ice cream parlor once in awhile as reward for your hard work and dedication to make a change. You can also set some goals to achieve for the week and set the reward for that goal. Keep doing this so you'll keep yourself motivated.

Find a partner in doing this change

Finding someone to remind you of your goals would be a great help to be successful in this change. If you are still starting out to practice waking up early, chances are you will find it hard to wake up and get up immediately. It would be best to find someone who has the goals as you are so you can both help each other in the process. Finding a partner who understands you or has the same goals as you can be your helping hand when you're having some difficulty waking up early in the morning.

Change Gradually

Becoming an early riser doesn't need to happen immediately. It is not advisable to make drastic changes in your schedule just so you can immediately see the results. If you make an extreme revamp, you'll definitely fail in your first attempt. Change gradually. Your body would have a hard time adapting to the change if it is too drastic or big. So, make a plan and assess your schedule. If you are used to waking up every 8am, then try to adjust the time and change it to 7:45am which is 15 minutes before your usual waking time. Although the change may seem too small, it actually helps as it allows your body to adapt slowly to these small changes. After you are comfortable with the new time, adjust it again and change it to 7:30am until you can set the time at 6am or 5:30am.

Record your progress

Keep a record of your progress. Make sure to have a notebook where you can track of your progress. Any improvement in your routine or adjustment in the time you wake up should be noted. This would help you see how far you've come and what you have achieved so far. Keeping a record of your progress would help you assess which area needs improvement and so you can plan your best action to improve.

Start Now

If you have been thinking of the best day or time to start rising early, make the decision now. Decide to become an early riser today so you can enjoy the amazing benefits of being an early riser. All you need is the determination and focus to achieve it. Although, it might be difficult at first because you need to set aside other things and break some of your habits, you will find it rewarding when you can achieve it. Along with the perks of being an early riser, you can also appreciate being one with the nature and would be grounded for few minutes.

Chapter 6 – Step By Step Guide: How to Be Productive in the Morning

As an early riser, one must know the importance of time. Of course, all your efforts will be wasted if you do not know what to prioritize and how to manage your time. The first thing you have to do is to list all the tasks you have to do daily, weekly, and monthly. If you have a specific project that needs to be done at a specific date, place it in a special column. Also, identify how many hours and how many days it will take you to finish the job. After listing, here's what you have to do.

"Difficult to Easy – Easy to Difficult" Dilemma

Some people are having difficulty managing their time because they do not know what to do first. Prioritizing tasks is an essential step to become productive day-by-day. Now, after you have written the master list of projects and tasks, assess each according to its complexity. (Is it difficult or easy?) Write 1 for Difficult and 2 for Easy. Now, separate those tasks that are urgent (has a deadline) and those following a routine. Arrange it in a project graph or you can also place the dates in an empty calendar.

When you are dealing with daily tasks, list them from the most urgent and most difficult task. Next is the most urgent and easy tasks, less urgent easy task, and last is the less urgent difficult task. Make a checklist of these tasks and mark each one that you have already finished. In this way, you will be able to finish all the tasks needed in a day.

Time Saving Tip

If you have free time like lunch and coffee breaks, you can check your mails or send important emails. These tasks are easy to do and can be finished within a few minutes.

Allot time for Each Task

The next thing you have to do is to allot a specific time frame for each task. You have to be very strict with your time and also be realistic. If it is too difficult, then allot an hour or two for it. Do not pressure yourself too much. You have the option to lengthen or shorten the time of each. It depends on you skill and ability to finish it.

Those are the tips you can use, as an early riser, in managing and prioritizing your time. If at first, you seem to fail to follow your schedule, don't despair. With practice you can eventually be a productive and efficient time manager.

Chapter 7 – A Future of Good Health

Did you know that there are 5 health benefits you stand to gain if you become an early riser? Since you are now living in a stress-free, organized, and energetic world – free from over fatigue and late night work – your body automatically rejuvenates and recovers from every day's workload.

1. Less Risk of Depression

Early risers have lower risk of depression because these people sleep early. In a study conducted in 2013 in Germany, they have found a high correlation between late sleeping and depression.

2. Consistency in Workouts

According to the study presented at the SLEEP 2014 by a group of Associated Professional Sleep Societies LLC, early birds have a lower tendency to blow off workouts. Night owls find it hard to find a fitness schedule and to stick to it. Also, they said that a person becomes sedentary when waking up late. This means, if you are an early riser, the more you can find time to jog or hit the gym than those who sleep late. You can now enjoy a healthy and fit body by just being an early riser.

3. In Control of Life

A study published the Journal of Applied Social Psychology last 2009 said that people who wake up early in the morning have larger goals and are proactive. They can confidently say "I can make this happen." Or "I can achieve big dreams." Also, these people are more organized. They monitor their work and take note of their goals.

4. Positive Outlook in Life and Cheerful

People who wake up early in the morning are more cheerful than those who wake up late. They also have a positive outlook in life. They see the downfall and mistakes as opportunities to improve. If something bad happened, they analyze the situation and focus on the lesson they learned from it. They do not spend so much time agonizing about the bad stuff.

5. Practices Healthy Eating

Early risers are more energetic than those who sleep late. That's why they do not indulge into eating fast food or chocolates. They have more control with what to eat. People who sleep late tend to:

- have higher average BMI

- Eat ½ less fruits and vegetables

- Twice as much fast food

- consumes 248 more calories

This is compared to early risers according to a Northwestern University study conducted last 2011.

So basically, sleeping late is abusing yourself and preventing your body from becoming healthy. Changing your daily routine and becoming an early riser will definitely help you become healthier and fitter than before. If you want to invest in a future of good health, you'd better start training yourself to sleep early and wake up early.

Chapter 8 – The Models: Prominent People Who Succeeded Because of Becoming an Early Riser

If you are still not convinced about the benefits of becoming an early riser, here are some prominent people from popular brands and a short description on how waking up early helped them succeed. This will serve as an inspiration for people who want to be an early riser for life.

Tim Cook, Apple CEO

According to Gawker's Ryan Tate, Mr. Cook tends to wake up around 4:30 AM to send company emails. And by 5AM, he usually works out in the gym. He is proud that he's the first one in the office and the last one to leave.

Bob Iger, Disney CEO

Mr. Iger wakes up around 4:30 AM, says the New York Times. He spends this quiet time to listen to music, exercise, watch TV, check emails and read papers. In his quiet time, he is also multitasking.

Howard Shultz, Starbucks CEO

According to Bloomberg BusinessWeek, Shultz said that he wakes up at 4:30AM to work out and walk his dogs. Also, he also makes coffee for himself and his wife using a Bodum French press. (8-Cup) Also, according to Portfolio.com, he gets to his office by 6AM.

Gerry Layborne, Former Oxygen Channel CEO

This former CEO will wake up by 6AM and will leave the house after 30 minutes. She said that, in a week she goes for a walk to connect with young people (youth) and to exercise. Also, she mentioned that doing this allows her to keep in touch with the next generation. Lastly, she said that people who wake up in the morning are serious about life. (According to Yahoo Finance) She enjoys the benefits of being an early riser.

A.G. Lafley, Procter & Gamble CEO

According to Fortune, A.G. Lafley makes it a habit to wake up around 5-5:30 AM and to sit in front of his desk by 6:30 to 7AM. Also, he said that, before, he didn't give breakfast much importance. But now, he makes sure that he has eaten any of the following: a cup of yoghurt, a V-8 juice, and half a bagel.

Conclusion

Thank you again for purchasing this book!

I hope this book was able to help you realize how amazing it would be to become an early riser. From keeping your body healthy and having you a clear mind, being an early riser paves the way to greater things.

It is also the best way to increase your productivity. Being productive doesn't need to be exhausting. You don't need to have plenty of tools to help you out in improving your productivity. All you need is yourself and the willingness to embrace the change that can lead you to become an early riser.

The next step is to put in action everything that you have read in this book. You may add some great ideas that you have in mind. I'm sure there are plenty of significant ideas that you would like to apply. All the information you have read in this book are helpful tips and boosters to keep you started, the rest is up to you.

With the right information and the determination to be more productive, becoming an early riser would be an enjoyable journey for you.

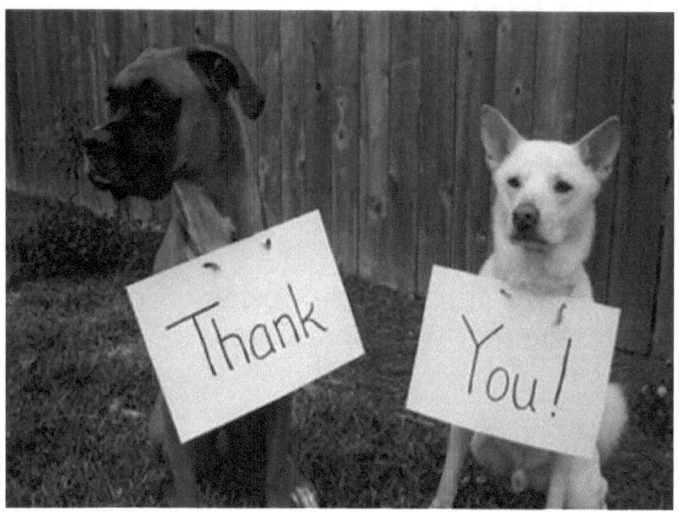

Finally, if you enjoyed this book, please take the time to share your thoughts and post a review on Amazon. It'd be greatly appreciated!

Thank you and good luck!

Check Out My Other Books

Below you'll find some of my other popular books that are popular on Amazon and Kindle as well. Simply click on the links below to check them out. Alternatively, you can visit my author page on Amazon to see other work done by me. If the links do not work, for whatever reason, you can simply search for these titles on the Amazon website to find them.

1) The Ultimate Guide To Overcome Anger - How To Manage Your Anger Before It Controls You

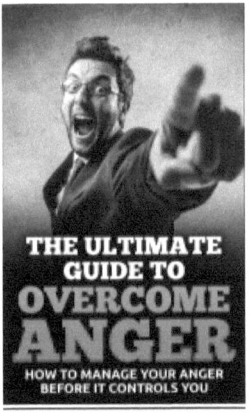

go to: http://amzn.to/1Pzm3Yy

2) The Ultimate Guide To Become An Alpha Male - How To Attract Women, Win In Life And Be Confident

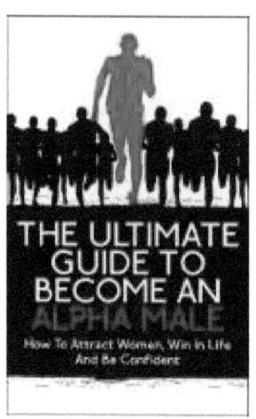

go to: http://amzn.to/20G8bB0

3) The Ultimate Guide To Overcome Porn Addiction For Life - The Most Effective, Permanent Solution To Finally Stop Porn Addiction

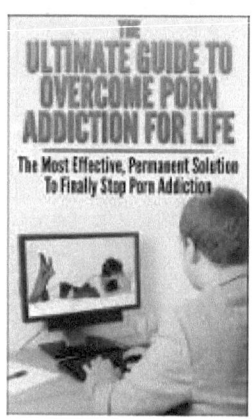

go to: http://amzn.to/1NZ2tmN

4) The Drug Addiction Cure - The Most Effective, Permanent Solution to Finally Overcome Drug Addiction for Life

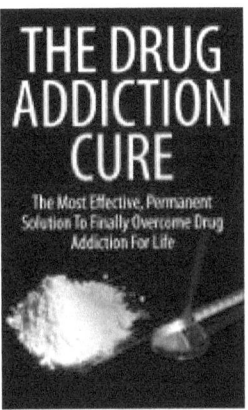

Or go to: http://amzn.to/1kkb9uc

5) How to Stop Snoring for Life - The Most Effective Cures and Remedies for Snoring

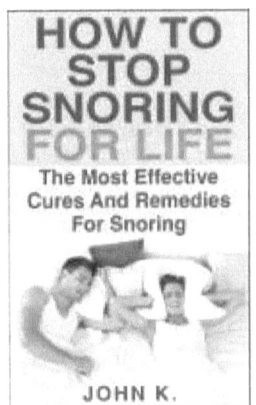

go to: http://amzn.to/1NE9uLn

www.ingramcontent.com/pod-product-compliance
Lightning Source LLC
Chambersburg PA
CBHW050525290526
45786CB00007B/2705